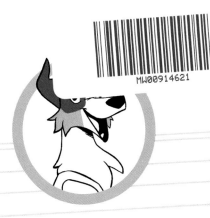

DASH CAN DO IT
Taking On Diabetes

By **PAT McCAW, M.D.**

Illustrated by **BETH HUGHES**

MAYO CLINIC PRESS KIDS

With gratitude to the Mayo Clinic Child Life Services Team

MAYO CLINIC PRESS KIDS | An imprint of Mayo Clinic Press
200 First St. SW
Rochester, MN 55905
mcpress.mayoclinic.org
To stay informed about Mayo Clinic Press, please subscribe to our free e-newsletter at mcpress.mayoclinic.org or follow us on social media.

For bulk sales to employers, member groups, and health-related companies, contact Mayo Clinic at SpecialSalesMayoBooks@mayo.edu.

Proceeds from the sale of every book benefit important medical research and education at Mayo Clinic.

ISBN: 978-1-945564-93-2 (paperback) | 978-1-945564-92-5 (library binding) | 978-1-945564-94-9 (ebook) | 979-8-88770-071-7 (multiuser PDF) | 979-8-88770-070-0 (multiuser ePub)

Library of Congress Control Number: 2022060867. Library of Congress Cataloging-in-Publication Data is available upon request.

TABLE OF CONTENTS

MEET DASH

"DAAASH-EEEE!"

Her voice pulls me from a happy dream. Half of me is still running through the woods with Blinky on my back. I'm playing tag with a whole forest of squirrels, gliding up and down tree trunks and nosing at their fluffy tails.

"Dash-girl, are you still napping?"

Hmph. The woods are fading away, and I'm back in my cozy bed in Navya's kitchen. *I'll be back, squirrels!*

"Are you ready, spaghetti?"

That's Navya. She's the very best human there is, and I love her with all my heart. She gave me her home, and this soft bed, and my pal Blinky here. I couldn't ask for more—except maybe ten more minutes of shut-eye.

I let out a sigh and open my heavy eyelids just enough to make out Navya's shape walking toward me. She's wearing her sneakers and carrying my—

"Let's go walk!" Navya says as she waves a black leash in my direction.

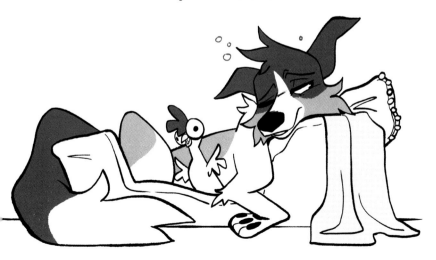

My eyes fly open and my legs spring into action, suddenly bursting with energy. *I'm up!* I sit still while Navya clips the leash to my collar.

Something is different about today. Usually, I wake up from my nap, have a drink of water, then run upstairs to tell Navya it's time for our walk. But today, Navya beat me to it. Not that I'm complaining—maybe we're going for an extra-long walk!

Navya bends down to pat the side of my belly. "Just a quick walk today, Dash," she says, reading my mind. "Today is your first day of work with me."

The hospital! That's right!

I leap outside as Navya opens the door to the backyard.

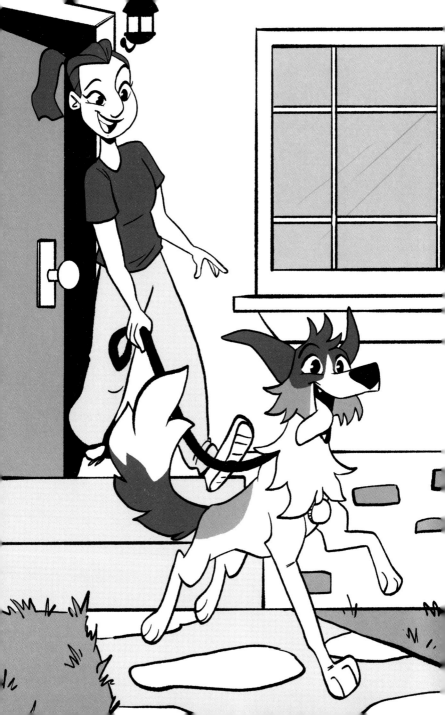

I can't believe I'd forgotten. I've been training at Helping Paws Academy for two years to learn how to help kids in the hospital. Last month, I was paired with Navya and finally became a certified facility dog. That means I work with Navya, who is a Certified Child Life Specialist (CCLS), to help kids learn about and feel comfortable at the hospital. And today is my first day on the job!

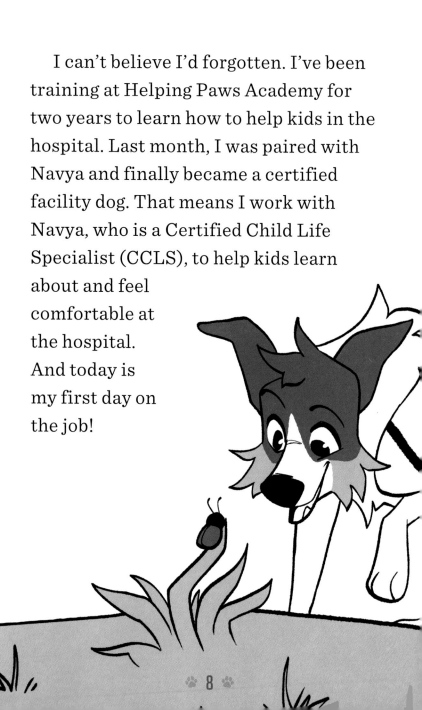

"Dash, let's go," Navya says as she gently pulls at my leash. I give the bug I found one last sniff. I can't help it. Bugs are so funny, the way they move like armored robots. Sniffing them is one of my favorite hobbies—that, and napping with Blinky.

"No time for bugs today," Navya says as we walk away from my new friend. *I'll be back, bug!*

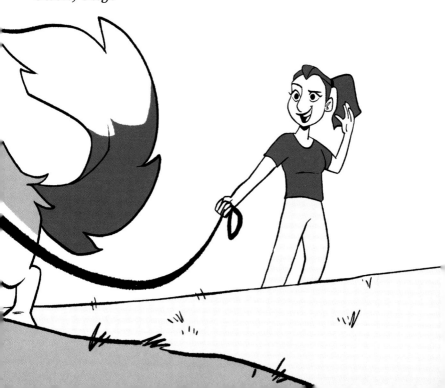

I sense Navya picking up her pace.

"Remember to stay focused on our work when we're at the hospital, Dash," she says.

Is Navya worried I won't be a good facility dog? Suddenly, my stomach starts to feel like it did the time I ate half a bag of treats when I was a puppy.

We turn back onto our street, and I see Navya's car waiting in the driveway. I feel my stomach turn over.

"You've got this, Dash," Navya says, sensing my uncertainty. "I believe in you."

I take a deep breath. If Navya believes in me, I can too!

After a bathroom break and a big drink of water, we're ready for the hospital. Navya wears a badge that shows she's a CCLS. She carries my uniform in one hand and opens the car door with the other. I take a running start and jump into the car.

"Good girl, Dash."

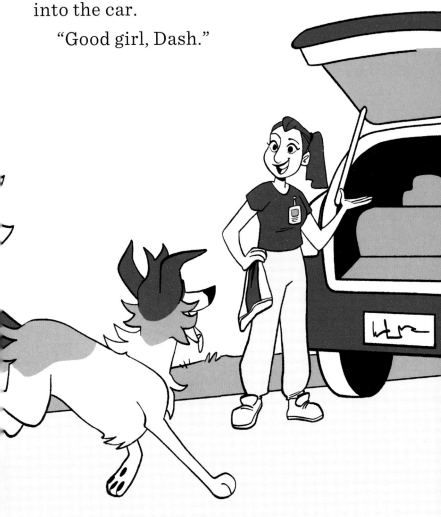

My name suits me because I love to run and play. But I learned throughout my training to be calm while I'm working. I sit still as Navya puts on my seat belt harness and secures it. Then I lick her nose for good measure.

Navya backs out of the driveway, and we're on the road. After a few minutes driving in silence, Navya glances at me in the rearview mirror and smiles.

"Almost there, pup."

The car slows as we approach a stop sign. Just outside, two kids run through a sprinkler in their yard. One of them shrieks with delight as the water hits him.

I can't help but stand up and wag my tail. I want to play too!

Navya's smiling eyes glance back at me through the mirror.

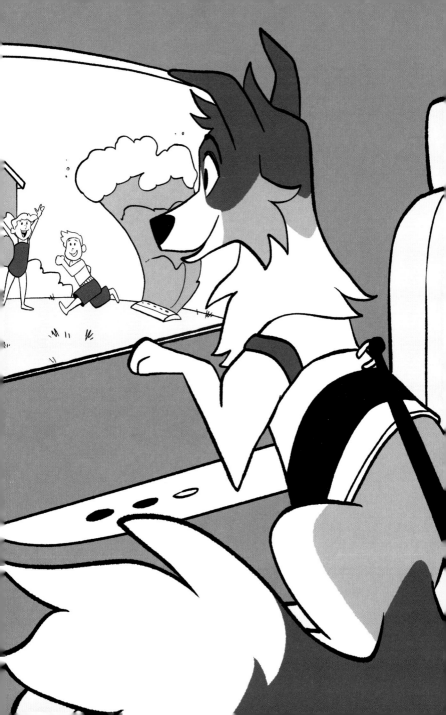

"I know you get excited when you see kids playing, Dash. But remember, there will be kids just like those at the hospital. They'll need you to be calm for them."
I raise my ears so Navya knows I understand.

A few minutes later, we pull into the hospital parking lot. Now I feel as though I've eaten a full bag of treats, including the bag.

Navya parks the car and removes my seat belt harness. "Time to put on your uniform," she says, holding out a blue vest with a patch that says Helping Paws. The uniform tells others, *I'm a working facility dog.*

My heart beats a little faster as I step into the vest and Navya clicks it in place. She stands back and looks at me with a smile. I love when she looks at me that way.

"Look at you, Dash-girl. You are so professional!"

The pride in Navya's voice makes me sit up a little taller. As I do, a familiar face catches my eye.

Hey, I know her!

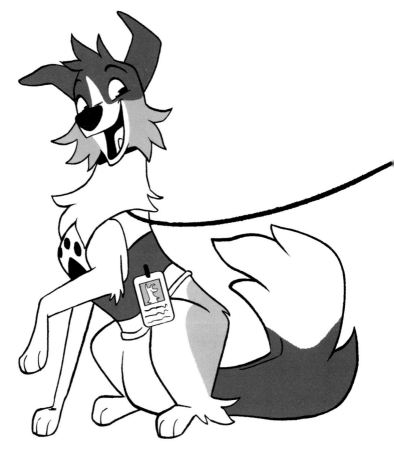

2

HOSPITAL HELPERS

"CRICKET!"

Walking toward Navya and me is a bubbly white Havanese with bouncing brown ears.

Now that I'm in uniform, I resist the urge to run toward my friend. Instead, I stand up and wag my tail to greet her.

I know Cricket from Helping Paws Academy. Soon after we met, we were *fur-ever* friends. But that's Cricket—she's easy to love. Now she's a facility dog like me. She started working at the hospital a few weeks ago.

Navya and I walk with Cricket and her handler, Tunde, toward the hospital entrance. On the way, I admit to Cricket that I'm feeling a little nervous.

"*Paw-lease!*" she says. "You're going to love every kid you meet!"

Seeing my friend is just the boost of confidence I need to walk through the doors.

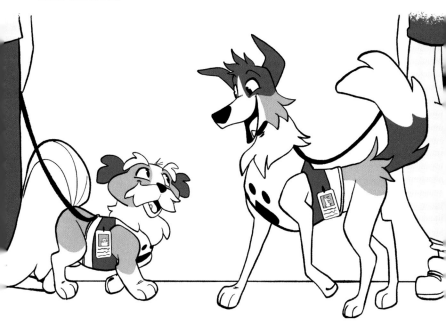

Inside the building, I can hardly believe my eyes. The atrium of the children's hospital is the most magical place! Colorful wooden birds hang from the high ceilings, their wings stretched out in flight. The walls are painted to look like a forest, the kind I was running through in my dream earlier this morning.

Best of all, there are kids—lots of them. Some are running, and some are curled up in the arms of parents. One is being pushed in a wheelchair, another pulled in a wagon.

While Navya signs into the computer to find out which patients we'll be seeing, I take it all in.

"It's great, isn't it?" Cricket says. "All these kids!"

I wag my tail. "I can't wait to play with them!"

Cricket hesitates. "Remember, Dash. Kids are here because they're sick or injured. They may not always be up to playing."

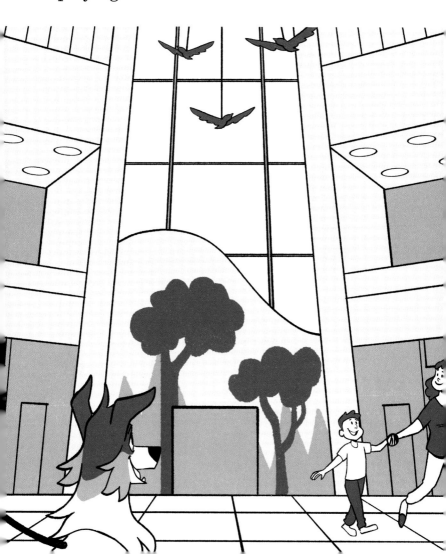

"Right," I say. "Of course. I didn't mean . . . I just meant . . ."

"I know what you meant," Cricket says, wagging her tail. "Don't worry, Dash. You'll be great!"

"Thanks, Cricket."

As I smile back at Cricket, her eyes jump to look at something behind me.

"Lumos!" she says.

Has Cricket already made friends with another facility dog? I turn around to see. Walking toward us is a wise-looking Golden Labrador and his handler. The woman wears a badge like Navya's, and it says her name is Eun Ji. The dog wears a Helping Paws vest like mine. He must have graduated from the academy long before I did!

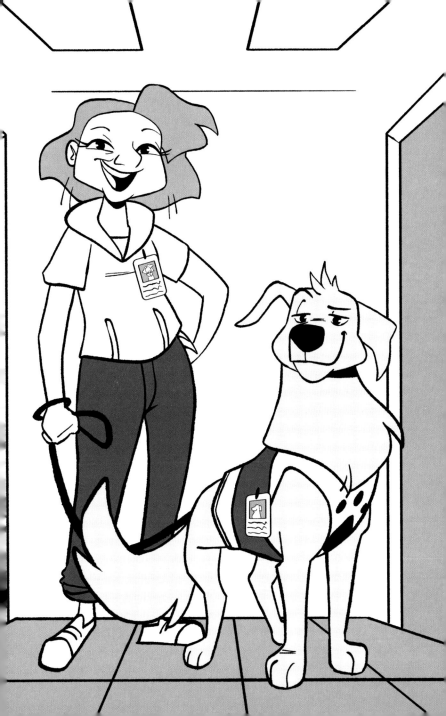

"Dash, this is Lumos," Cricket says, looking fondly at the Golden Labrador. "Lumos is a certified facility dog like us. But he's been working here for more than two years!"

Lumos nods to acknowledge Cricket's introduction, and I manage a squeaky "Hello." Lumos looks serious, like he's never snuck into a bag of treats in his life.

The confidence I felt with Cricket begins to wane in Lumos's presence.

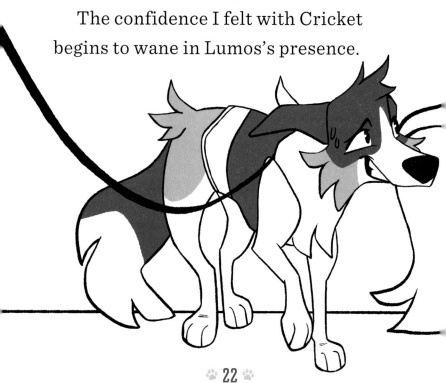

He knows so much, and I know so little! Next to him, I'm just a rookie who can't sleep without her blue chicken.

As Lumos walks off, I hear Navya's voice above me.

"Okay, Dash-girl, we're all set."

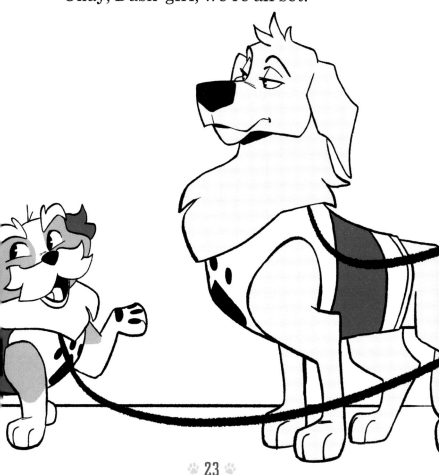

3

THE FIRST PATIENT

"WE'RE HEADING TO FLOOR TWO, DASH" NAVYA SAYS AS she presses the Up arrow by the elevator. She carries a printed-off list of the patients we're going to visit. I can tell we have a busy day ahead of us. I wish I felt as calm and collected as Navya looks!

The elevator doors open and we step inside. I turn to face the closing doors and sit, trying to look professional for Navya. I wonder how Lumos sits in an elevator. Does he look straight ahead, or up at his handler?

Navya pets my head. "Our first stop is with a patient named Francisco. He's ten years old."

Francisco! Ten years old! I can't help but grin. After two years of training, I'm finally meeting a real patient.

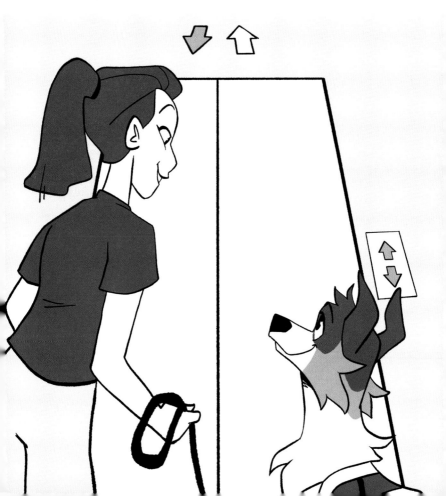

The elevator doors open to reveal floor two. Francisco is here, somewhere, waiting for me.

"Ready, Dash-girl?"

I stand tall to show Navya that I am. Navya takes a deep breath, and we step out into the second-floor hall. After glancing at the paper in her hand, she makes a right turn, and we set off down the hall. On our way, I hear the voices of kids floating from the rooms we pass. One child cheers "Puppy!" as we walk by. I want so badly to stop and say hello, but I keep walking. Francisco is waiting!

Navya begins to slow her pace, looking from the paper in her hand to the door we are approaching. This must be it.

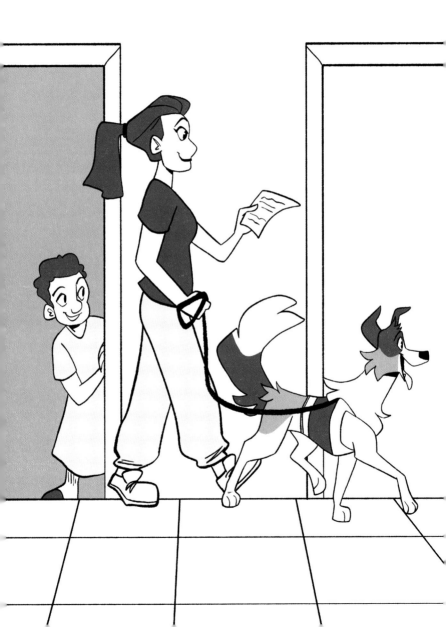

As we approach the door, a woman with curly brown hair and shiny hoop earrings steps out of the room. She wears a white coat with an ID badge hanging on it.

"Navya, hello!" the woman says.

"Hi, Dr. Lopez," Navya says, and she gestures to me. "This is Dash, the newest member of our team. She's a facility dog who works with me."

"Good to meet you, Dash!" Dr. Lopez says.

Navya glances over Dr. Lopez's shoulder at the partially open room door. "We're here to see Francisco."

"I'm glad you're here," Dr. Lopez nods. "Francisco's been diagnosed with type 1 diabetes. He's staying at the hospital while we get his blood sugar back to within typical range and start his treatment routines." She glances back at the room door before continuing, her voice lower.

"He hasn't said much in the last couple of hours. I think a visit from you and Dash would be good for him."

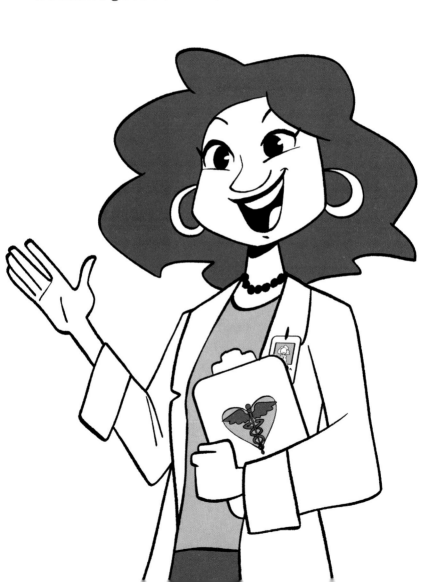

What are we waiting for? I want to shout. *This is why I'm here!*

I sit up a little straighter, showing Dr. Lopez that I'm ready to help. She notices my movement and squats down to look me in the eyes. "Maybe you can help us, Dash."

Dr. Lopez knocks twice on the door as she pushes it back open. Inside, a boy sits up in his bed. His eyes look weary.

"Francisco, this is Navya and Dash. They're here to talk with you about how they can support you in the hospital."

I lock eyes with Francisco. A faint smile lifts his cheeks and lights up his eyes. All the nerves and doubts I felt five minutes ago are suddenly gone. All I feel is love for Francisco.

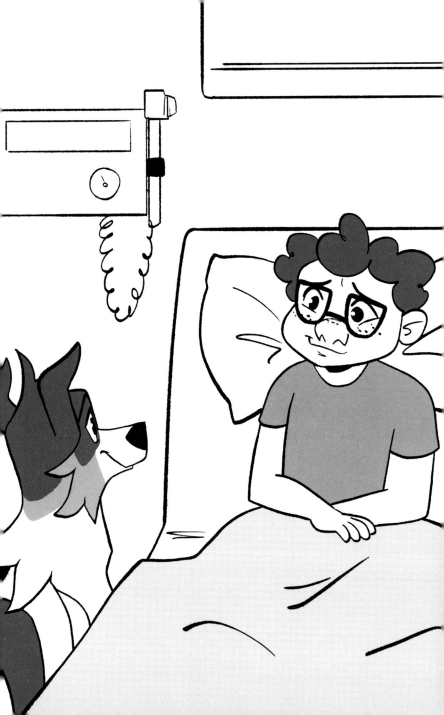

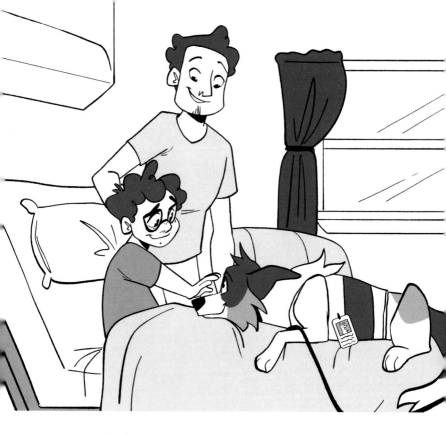

"Would you like her to join you in your bed?" Navya asks. Francisco nods, and Navya pats the bed. "Jump, Dash."

I hop up on the bed and settle in at Francisco's feet.

"You made a new friend, huh, Pancho?" The voice comes from a man I hadn't noticed when I walked in.

"I'm Francisco's dad," the man says to Navya. "Andres."

Francisco and his dad have the same soft brown eyes. My muscles relax under their kind smiles. I rest my chin on Francisco's foot, and he pats me on the head.

Am I comforting Francisco, or is he comforting me?

"Do you mind if we stay with you for a bit, Francisco?" Navya asks. "We could learn a little more about you and maybe help you learn about what's going on in your body."

Andres smiles at Francisco, who nods quietly as he gives my nose a pat.

4

FRANCISCO'S STORY

AS FRANCISCO SCRATCHES MY EARS, ANDRES explains to Navya that Francisco hadn't been feeling well for the past few weeks. During his soccer games, he wanted to go after the ball, but he couldn't find the energy. His head hurt and his legs were heavy. When he and Andres went to see a movie, he missed all the best parts because he had to take a bathroom break every twenty minutes. That's when Andres knew something wasn't right.

Navya turns to Francisco. "There is an organ in your body called the pancreas. Its job is to make insulin. Insulin helps turn glucose, or sugar, from food and drinks you eat into energy to do all the things you enjoy, like soccer. Sometimes the pancreas stops making insulin. It's no one's fault; it just happens. And without insulin, your body has not been getting energy. That's why you feel tired."

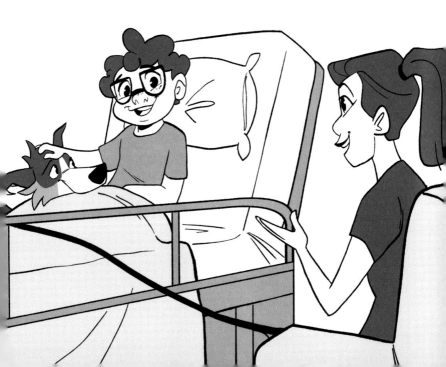

"Meanwhile," Dr. Lopez says, "your body was trying to get rid of the extra glucose in your blood by peeing. That's why you had to go to the bathroom so much."

I look up at Francisco, trying to read how he's feeling. He slowly nods but doesn't say a word. Instead, he gazes past me, like he'd rather be anywhere but here, learning about his diabetes.

What can I do? I'm only a dog. *But*, I remind myself, *that's why I'm here: to be a dog.*

Navya catches my eye and smiles as she gives the command. I roll onto my back, exposing my belly. A quiet laugh escapes Francisco's mouth, as I suspected it would. Humans seem to love when I do this.

"Dash loves belly rubs," Navya tells Francisco.

"So do I!" Andres jokes, reaching over to scratch my belly. I knew I liked this guy.

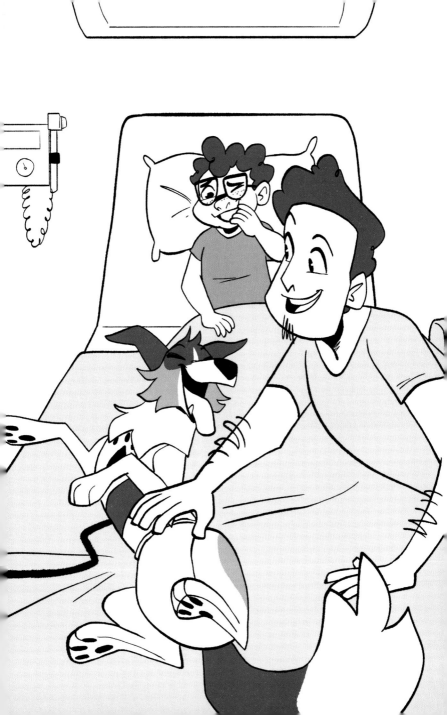

Francisco lightly pats me at first, unsure exactly how it's done. I give him my biggest grin to indicate that there's no wrong way to rub a belly. A smile on his face, Francisco now scratches up and down my belly. I try my best not to drool.

After the humans calm down from the belly-rubbing excitement, Dr. Lopez turns back to her patient.

"The good news, Francisco, is you can still do all the things you love—like play soccer, ride your bike, and eat ice cream sometimes. You'll just start some new routines to take care of your body."

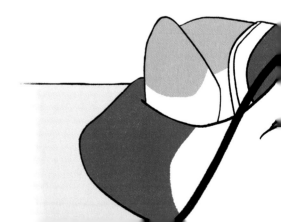

Francisco shifts in his bed, bending his knees up toward his chin. His eyes look weary again, like he's been dreading this part. I settle back in by his shins. *I'm right here, pal.*

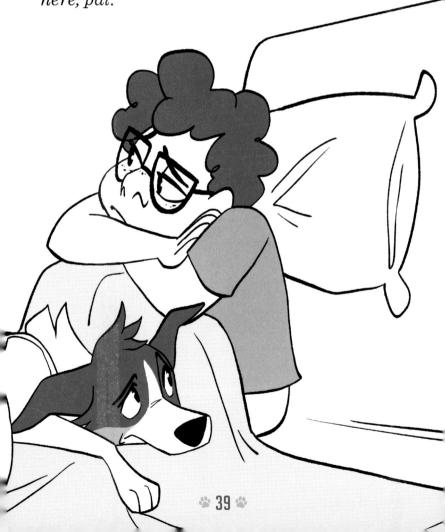

"You'll check your blood sugar before you eat meals or snacks," Dr. Lopez continues. "This will help you figure out how much insulin your body needs to turn the food you're eating into energy."

"Does it matter what type of food he eats?" Andres asks.

Dr. Lopez nods. "Foods that are high in carbohydrates, like pizza and pasta, require more insulin."

Francisco's brow furrows in confusion. "Don't worry," Dr. Lopez smiles. "You'll get the hang of all of this. And you'll have plenty of help. When you're at school, you'll go to the nurse's office to check your blood and get insulin."

Navya nods. "And you might find there are other kids at your school who need insulin shots too."

At the word *shots*, Francisco brings his knees close to his body and buries his face in his arms.

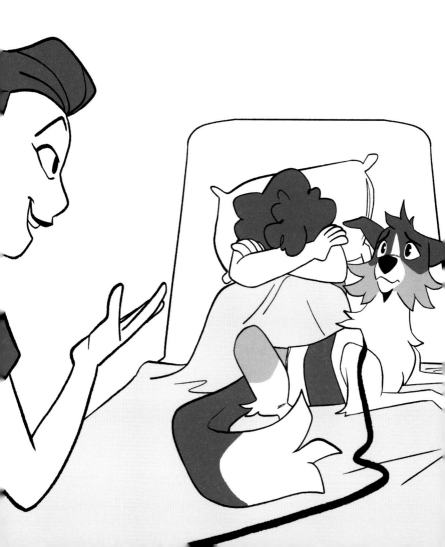

"I wonder how you might be feeling right now, Francisco," Navya says warmly.

Andres sits down on the edge of the bed and places his hand gently over the back of Francisco's head. "He's always had a hard time with needles," Andres responds.

"Other kids do too, Francisco," Navya says. "Shots can be hard. Even though getting pokes isn't a choice, there are some choices you can make about how you get them."

"I know it's a lot, Pancho," Andres says. "And it's okay to feel everything you're feeling. But there is a whole team of people here who are going to help us learn everything we need to know."

Just then, I see Cricket pass by in the hallway, followed by Tunde. *Are they already moving on to their next patient?*

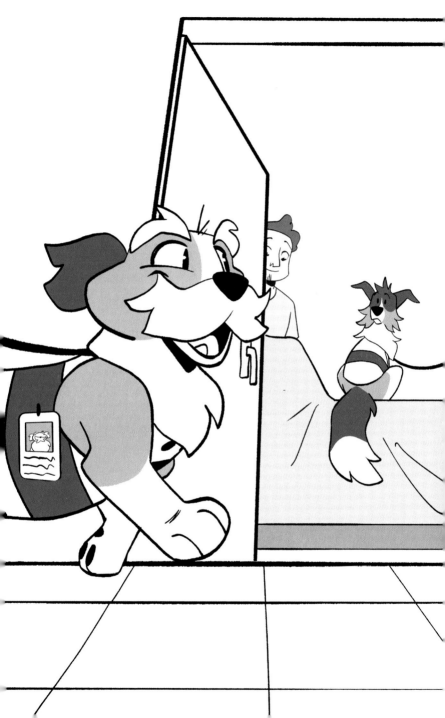

I turn to Navya, wondering what to do next.

"Francisco," Navya says, "we can take a break from this tough talk for now. Is that okay with you? Dash and I have some other kids to see."

I sit up to face Francisco and look him in the eye. I want to tell him everything will be okay. He looks back at me for a moment. Then he crosses his ankles, leans forward, and wraps his arms around me.

"You'll come back?" For a moment, I'm not sure who asked the question. Francisco's voice is quiet and raspy, like he hasn't spoken in hours.

Andres is fighting back tears. Dr. Lopez looks relieved to hear Francisco speak. She looks over to Navya. "Maybe you could stop back after you visit the other patients?"

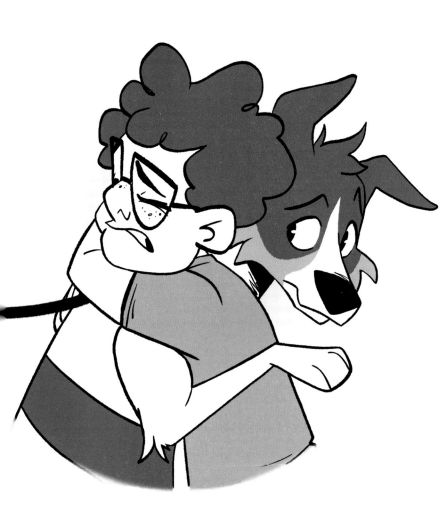

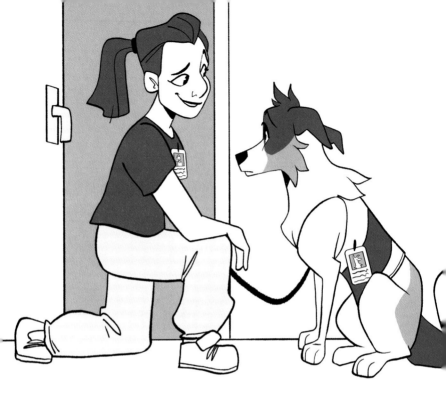

Navya closes Francisco's door behind us as we step back into the hall. I try not to whimper as I look back at his room. Navya sees that I'm sad to leave Francisco. She bends down on one knee and scratches the top of my head.

"You did such a good job with your first patient, Dash," she says, holding my chin in her palm. "Francisco really liked you."

I look down at the floor, then back at Francisco's door.

"I know you really liked him too. We'll come back to see him before we leave. But for now, we have other patients to help."

I lock eyes with Navya. I know she'll make sure we see Francisco again.

5

AN IDEA FROM LUMOS

"OUR NEXT STOP IS SIX-YEAR-OLD LENA," NAVYA SAYS, standing up. "She's on the fourth floor. Let's take the stairs this time. We're running behind, and I don't want to wait for an elevator."

We take off at a quick pace. I'm happy to take the stairs. It'll help me let out some of this energy in my legs. I think of Francisco feeling tired on the soccer field, his body low on energy.

As Navya opens the door to the stairwell, I look back toward Francisco's room.

"Let's go, Dash-ee. We're late!"

The stairwell is empty. Navya takes the stairs two at a time as I run alongside her. By the time we reach floor four, we're both out of breath. It feels so good to run!

"Good girl, Dash!" Navya scratches my chin. "Back to calm."

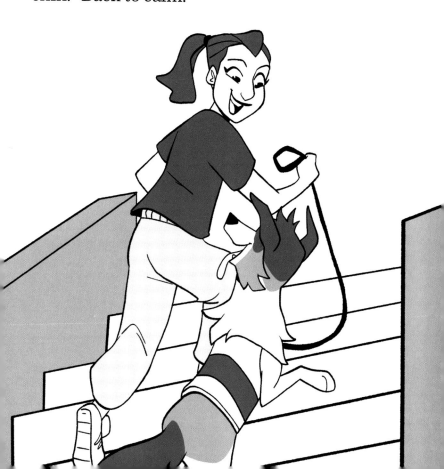

Navya opens the stairwell door. As we step onto the fourth floor, we nearly walk into Lumos. He's strolling alongside a patient who looks about Francisco's age. The patient moves slowly, like she's recovering from surgery. Lumos matches her pace.

"Hi, Lumos," I squeak, my voice higher than usual. But he doesn't turn my way.

Navya gently pulls me in the opposite direction. "Lena's this way."

As we walk toward Lena's room, I feel embarrassed for saying hi to Lumos. He was with a patient—he needed to stay focused! I hope he isn't upset with me.

"What's up, Dash?" Navya's voice breaks through my thoughts. "You look distracted."

I turn to face Navya and sit down, my head held high. I look her in the eyes to show I'm focused now.

"That's better." She gives me a
quick pat before knocking on the door
to Lena's room.

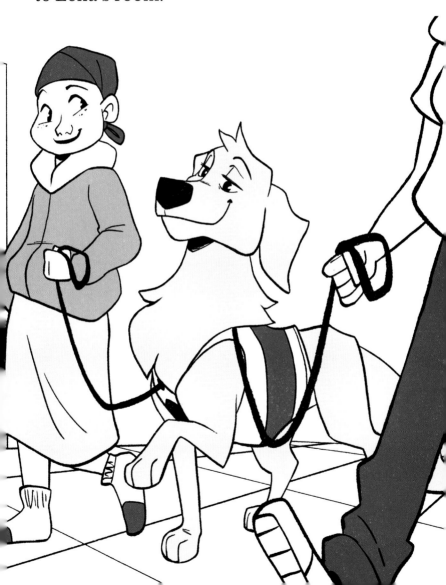

The next couple of hours are a blur of patients, family members, and doctors. There is Lena, who took me on a short walk. There is Leo, who put together a puzzle with me. And there is Jordan, who wanted nothing more than to nap with me. I wonder if he played tag with squirrels in his dream too!

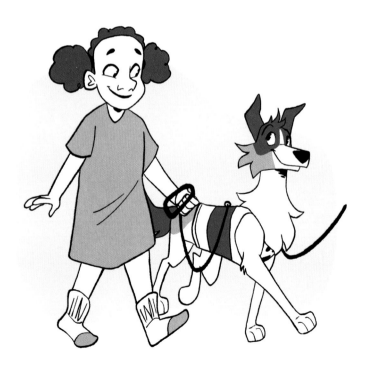

After every patient, I thought about Francisco. Now that we've visited all the patients on the list, I could really use a nap. But I still want to see Francisco one more time. I just don't know what I can do for him.

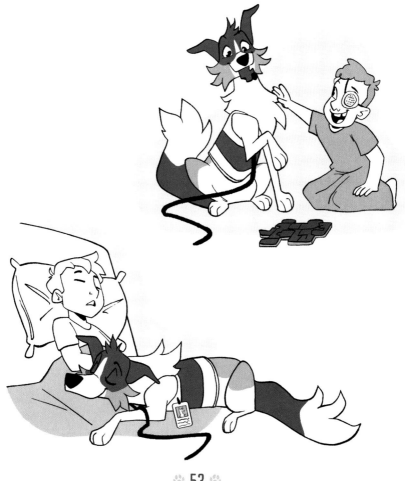

Navya and I make our way back to the second floor to see Francisco. This time we take the elevator. Navya pushes the Down arrow and stifles a yawn. The day was tiring for her, too, working with so many patients. She's a pretty great human.

As we wait for the elevator to arrive, I hear my name behind me.

"Hi, Dash."

I turn around to see Lumos and Eun Ji. Lumos is looking right at me.

"Hi—hi, Lumos," I sputter nervously.

"Sorry I couldn't talk before," he says. "I get really focused when I'm with a patient."

"Oh, that's okay," I say, rubbing my nose with a paw. "I shouldn't have said anything."

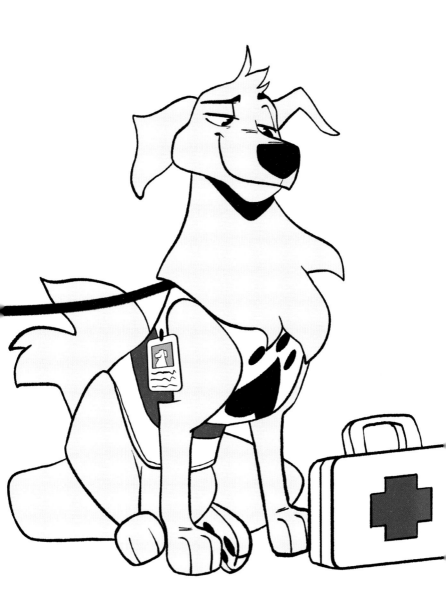

"Nonsense!" Lumos responds. "You can always say hi."

Our elevator arrives, and Navya waves goodbye to Lumos and Eun Ji. Before I turn to go, I notice a play medical kit sitting at Lumos's feet. He's probably going to bring the kit to a patient. I learned in training that medical play can help kids learn about their own procedures and treatments.

Now Navya is holding the elevator door open for me. "We have to go, Dash!" she says. I hop on the elevator and look back at my new friend. *Is he my new friend?*

"See you around, Dash," Lumos says. "Keep up the good work."

Yep. I have a new friend.

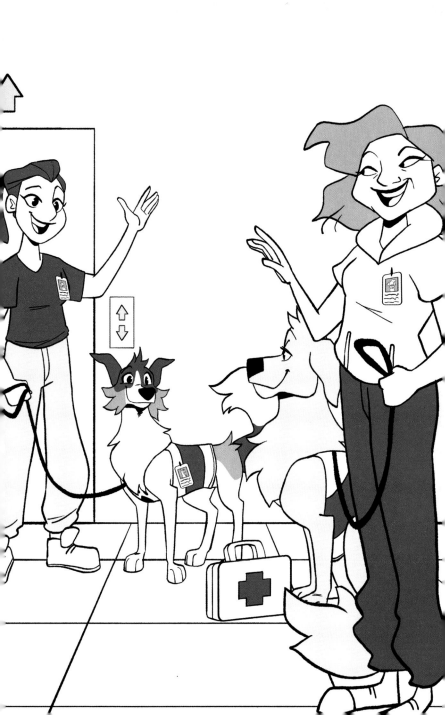

Riding down on the elevator, I think about Lumos's play medical kit. It gives me an idea for how I could help Francisco learn about his diabetes treatment.

I look up at Navya. She's deep in thought. After a moment, she looks back at me.

"You know, Dash," she says, her eyes still peering into her imagination. "That medical play kit Lumos had . . . it gives me an idea."

I grin at Navya. Every dog should get a human who can read her mind.

Back on the second floor, we find Francisco's room door partially open. I'm relieved to hear Andres's voice inside.

Part of me worried that Francisco left
while I was visiting other patients.

Now, Navya clutches a medical play
kit like the one Lumos had. "Knock,
knock," she says, announcing our arrival
outside Francisco's door.

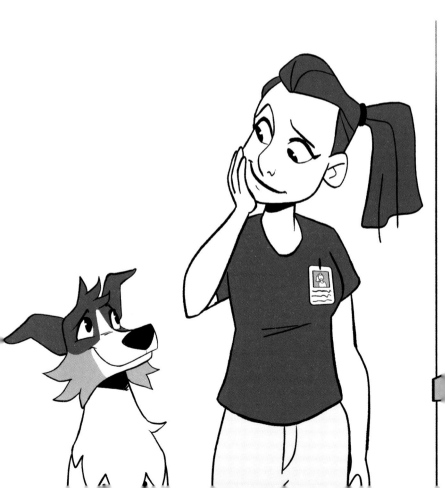

6

PATIENT DASH

"HI, DASH!" FRANCISCO LIGHTS UP WHEN HE SEES ME.
There's no better feeling.

"Hey, you came back!" Andres says, his eyes bright like Francisco's and a note of surprise in his voice. "We weren't sure you'd be able to fit us in."

"Of course we came back," Navya responds. "Dash insisted that we do."

Hearing this, Francisco smiles and extends his arms, inviting me onto his bed.

"Jump, Dash," Navya says.

I leap up, and Francisco throws his arms around me. Not all dogs like hugs, but I can't get enough of them! I don't even bother removing the silly grin from my face.

Just then, Dr. Lopez walks in.

"Aha!" she says. "You made it back! We weren't sure if we'd see you again."

I look at Francisco, my grin large as ever. *Humans. Don't they know how friendship works?*

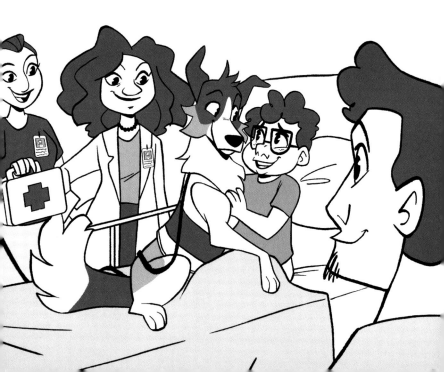

As I curl up by Francisco, Navya shows Francisco the medical play kit she brought.

"Dash and I want to help you learn about what to expect when you get pokes," she says. Francisco nods, and I sit up on the bed, ready to take orders.

"First things first, Dash," Navya says as she approaches the bed. "Let's check your blood sugar. Francisco, which paw do you think Dash would like to use?"

Francisco taps my right paw, and Navya extends her hand. "Shake, Dash," she says, and I happily give her my paw. "If Dash had diabetes," Navya explains, pointing to my wrist, "we'd give her paw pad a poke."

Navya pulls a play syringe from the medical kit. "Let's pretend this is a lancet, which is used to get just a drop or two of blood. Dash, your job is to hold your body still like a statue."

I lick my lips to show her I'm ready.

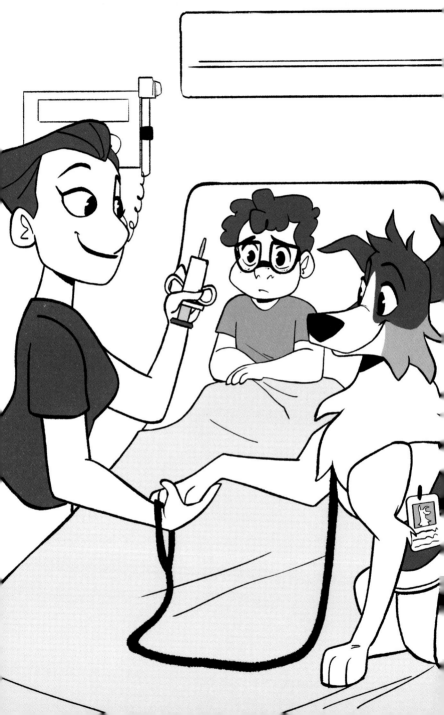

"First we use an alcohol wipe to clean Dash's skin," Navya explains to Francisco. "The wipe feels cold and wet. Then comes the poke. Dash can choose to count to three, sing a song, or take a deep breath. What do you think Dash would like to do?"

Francisco thinks for a moment. "Dash would like to count to three," he responds.

"Okay," Navya says. "One, two, three." She gently taps my paw pad with the play syringe. "The poke is done and the needle is out. Now we have a small drop of blood that we can test."

Francisco pats my back. "Good girl, Dash," he says.

"We put the drop of blood on a strip that tells the blood glucose meter how much glucose, or sugar, is in your body," Navya continues. "Let's say Dash's blood glucose level is at 300. That's a little high."

"Dash, your body needs insulin,"
Francisco tells me.

"That's right," Navya agrees. "Do you
think Dash wants the insulin shot in her
arm or leg?"

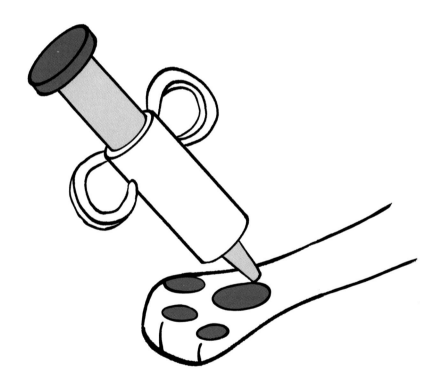

"Her arm," Francisco responds.

"And do you think she wants to be sitting or lying down?"

Francisco chooses for me to stay sitting up, and Navya gives the command.

Happy to!

Navya hands the play syringe to Francisco. "Will you give Dash her shot?"

Francisco nods and take the syringe. Navya points to my arm. "Right in her arm, like she chose."

I sit still as stone. Francisco cleans my fur with an alcohol wipe, then counts to three and gives me a pretend shot.

"Good job, Dash!" Navya says as Francisco beams at me. "You did a great job sitting still. You were very brave."

Andres rests a hand on his son's shoulder. "I know you can be brave like Dash, Pancho," he says.

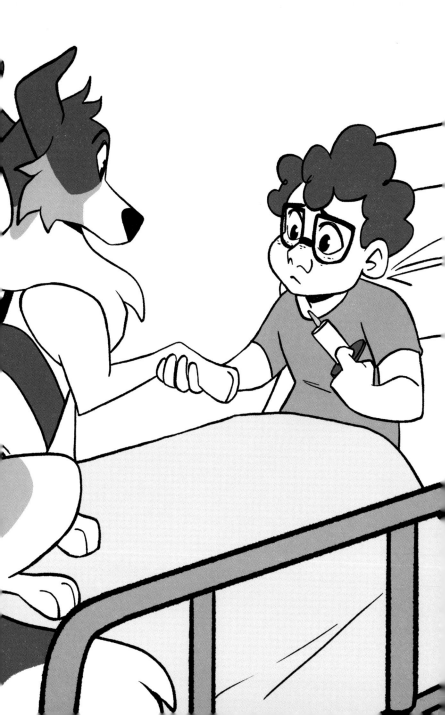

"Dash doesn't like needles either,"
Navya tells Francisco. "That's why we
take a few deep breaths and count to three
before a shot."

"That's a great way to stay calm,"
Dr. Lopez nods. "And maybe one day you'll
choose to use an insulin pump, which
delivers insulin to your body throughout
the day. That way you don't have to give
yourself daily injections."

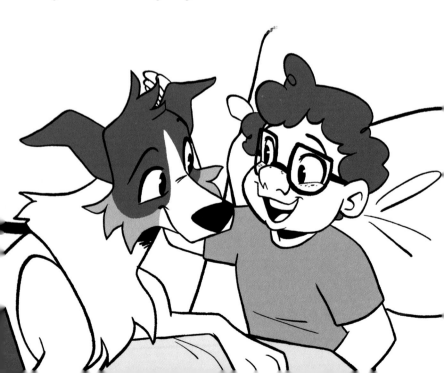

Francisco nods toward me. "Can dogs like Dash use insulin pumps?"

Dr. Lopez smiles. "That's a good question. Insulin pumps aren't as practical for dogs as they are for humans. But scientists are always researching new solutions for diabetes treatment, in both dogs and humans."

I look up at Francisco. He's no longer the weary boy that I met this morning.

"You hear that, Dash?" Francisco whispers, his eyes alive and determined. "We'll keep learning."

7

GOING HOME

NAVYA AND I STEP THROUGH THE HOSPITAL DOORS INTO the afternoon sunlight. I blink, remembering there's a world outside the children's hospital. I think of the dog I was when I arrived this morning—nervous, uncertain, and full of doubt. A lot has changed in the last few hours.

In the parking lot, we pass by Cricket as she and Tunde leave for the day.

"How'd your first day go, Dash?" Cricket shouts.

"You were right," I shout back. "It was great!"

Cricket laughs, then hops into the back seat of her car.

On the ride home, I think about Francisco. I was sad to say goodbye to him. But I'm glad he'll soon be leaving the hospital and getting back to his life. Navya's eyes smile at me from the rearview mirror.

"You were a natural today, buddy," she says. I wag my tail in gratitude.

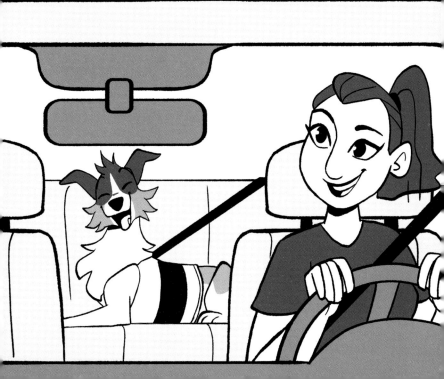

Back home, Navya pours a scoop of kibble into my dish. Then she heats up her leftovers from last night's dinner. *Bon appétit!* We chow down, too hungry and sleepy to pause for chatter.

After our dinner, my legs automatically carry me to my bed for my post-meal nap. There's Blinky, right where I left her. I pause, thinking of Lumos. I wonder if he has a naptime friend too.

Blinky looks back at me with her goofy bug eyes. *What are you waiting for?* she seems to say.

I climb into my soft bed and curl myself around her. *I may be a facility dog*, I tell her, *but that doesn't mean I don't need you.*

With Blinky under my chin, I drift off to sleep. In my dream, a ten-year-old boy with bright brown eyes scores the winning goal for his soccer team.

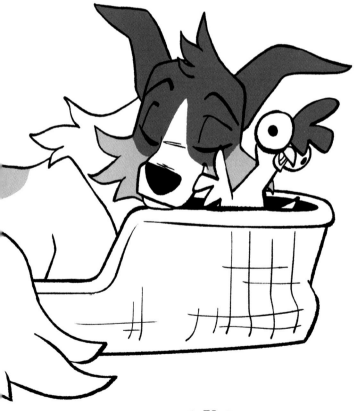

A Note from Francisco:
MORE ABOUT DIABETES

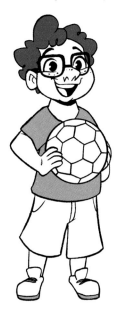

HI, READER! IT'S FRANCISCO, BUT YOU CAN CALL ME
Pancho. Want to know more about
diabetes? Well, you've come to the right
place; since being diagnosed, I've become a
bit of an expert!

Diabetes is a disease that affects how
my body manages glucose, or sugar.
The amount of sugar in a person's blood

increases when they eat food. Then their pancreas makes insulin, which helps sugar in the blood move into the body's cells. But because I have type 1 diabetes, my pancreas can't make insulin. (Some people have type 2 diabetes, which means their bodies don't respond to insulin or don't produce enough of it. But kids like me are more commonly diagnosed with type 1 diabetes.)

I went to the hospital showing symptoms of diabetes, like thirst, tiredness, and having to pee a lot. Dr. Lopez did some blood tests and found that I had high blood sugar. These tests confirmed that I have diabetes. Now, I work with Dr. Lopez to manage my disease with a treatment plan. This includes taking insulin shots to keep my blood sugar at normal levels. Every day I learn more about how to stay healthy so I can do all the things I love.

A Note from Dash:
MORE ABOUT FACILITY DOGS

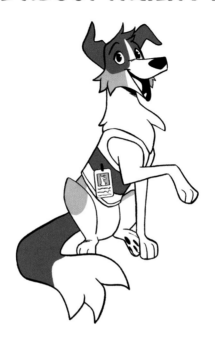

HELLO, FRIEND! DASH HERE. SINCE BECOMING A facility dog, I've been telling all my two- and four-legged pals about it. I'd love to tell you too!

Facility dogs like me are specially trained to work at a certain facility, such as a hospital or other healthcare setting, where we offer physical and emotional support to adults and children. We respond to more than forty commands to motivate patients and help them work toward their goals. Facility dogs are considered full-time workers, and their handlers are facility employees.

If you'd like to learn more about facility dogs, check out the websites below. And hey, thanks for reading!

Canine Companions—What Are the Differences Between Service Dogs, Facility Dogs, Therapy Dogs and Emotional Support Animals?

https://canine.org/service-dogs/service-dog-month/service-dog-differences/

Pet Partners—Terminology

https://petpartners.org/learn/terminology/

MEET ALICIA!

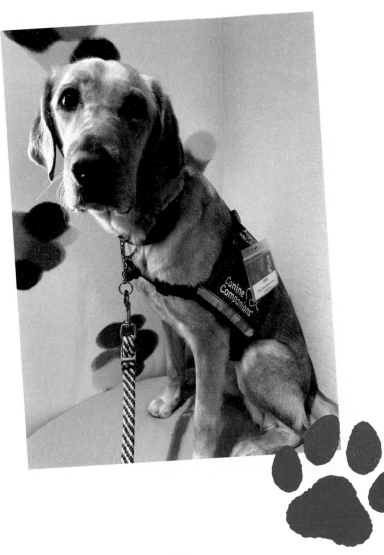

ALICIA IS THE FACILITY DOG AT MAYO CLINIC

Children's Center. The Golden Labrador was expertly trained from birth to two years old at Canine Companions. She works directly with her handler, Amy, CCLS, and their patient population.

Together, Amy and Alicia support patients' physical and psychological needs throughout their hospital stays. Alicia provides comfort during non-sterile procedures and motivation during treatment and recovery. She also takes part in medical play to help young patients understand and cooperate with their treatments or procedures.

At Mayo Clinic Children's Center, pediatric experts diagnose and treat all types of diseases and disorders in children. Specialists from different areas work as a team to find answers, set goals, and develop a treatment plan tailored to every child's needs.

READ ALL THE BOOKS IN THE HELPING PAWS ACADEMY SERIES!

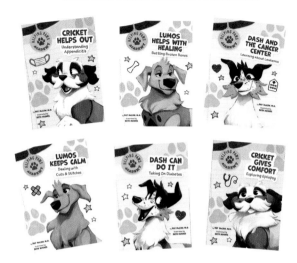

PAT McCAW, M.D., IS A FAMILY PRACTICE PHYSICIAN AND CHILDREN'S AUTHOR from Eldridge, Iowa. She is passionate about using books to help children with emotional and health issues. In addition to writing, she practices family medicine part-time and is a faculty physician at a medical residency program. Pat teaches classes on how to use picture books in the classroom and writes online educational lessons on science and physiology. If she has any free time, she loves to hike and fish while spending time with her family. Her dog, Poppy, rules the household. Pat's website and blog is found at www.patmccawauthor.com.